EVERYTHING ABOUT FABRY DISEASE

A Complete Guide For Patients, Caregivers, And Healthcare Professionals - Causes, Symptoms, Diagnosis, Treatment, Coping Strategies, And More

DR. CADE JOSUE

Table of Contents

DISCLAIMER

The information provided in this book is for general informational purposes only. It is not intended as medical advice, diagnosis, or treatment.

The content of this book should not be considered a substitute for professional medical advice. Readers should consult with a qualified healthcare provider for diagnosis and treatment of any medical conditions they have.

While every effort has been made to ensure the accuracy and completeness of the information presented, the author makes no representations or warranties of any kind, express or implied, about the completeness, accuracy, reliability, suitability, or availability with respect to the information, contained in this book.

The author disclaims any responsibility for any loss or damage resulting from reliance on the information provided in this book. References to individuals, products, websites, organizations, or other names are for informational purposes only and do not imply endorsement.

By reading this book, readers acknowledge that they are responsible for their own health decisions and should seek appropriate medical advice when necessary.

ABOUT THIS BOOK

This book titled "Everything About Fabry Disease" offers a comprehensive analysis of a rare genetic disorder that has far-reaching consequences for affected individuals and their families. The detailed table of contents of this book demonstrates its comprehensive nature, as it encompasses critical elements ranging from fundamental comprehension of the disease to more advanced subjects such as emergent therapies and holistic wellness methodologies.

The introduction provides an overview of Fabry's disease, establishing the foundation for a more comprehensive exploration of its complexities. The overview section explores the mechanisms, genetic underpinnings, and physiological effects of the disease across multiple bodily systems. A greater understanding of the factors that contribute to the development and progression of Fabry disease enables the formulation of more effective preventative measures and causes and risk factors.

This book comprehensively addresses indicators and manifestations, which are critical for prompt identification and diagnosis, before delving into an in-depth critique of diagnostic techniques and testing protocols. A comprehensive evaluation is conducted on treatment alternatives, encompassing pain management techniques and enzyme replacement therapy, to furnish clinicians and patients with invaluable knowledge regarding the efficient management of the disease's symptoms.

Furthermore, this book encompasses complications of the cardiovascular, renal, neurological, and dermatological systems in addition to medical interventions. With an emphasis on a holistic approach to treatment, management strategies tailored for children, genetic counseling, and the emotional impact on patients and families are also extensively covered.

Moreover, this book expands its scope to encompass more extensive factors, including financial implications, advocacy efforts, coping mechanisms, and improvements to quality of life. Additionally, this book explores current advancements in clinical trials, research, and teamwork among healthcare professionals, contributing to a holistic comprehension of Fabry disease management.

By emphasizing patient empowerment, education, and comprehensive problem-solving, this book functions as an indispensable reference for healthcare practitioners, patients, caregivers, and individuals in search of a nuanced comprehension of Fabry disease and its complex treatment.

CHAPTER ONE

Introduction

Fabry disease is an uncommon hereditary disorder distinguished by the insufficiency or nonexistence of alpha-galactosidase A (α-GAL A), an enzyme. The consequence of this insufficiency is the buildup of specific lipid compounds, predominantly globotriaosylceramide (GL-3 or Gb3), within the cellular structure of the entire organism.

As time passes, this accumulation has the potential to induce gradual harm to numerous organs and systems, culminating in an array of symptoms and complications.

A Synopsis Of Fabry Disease

Fabry disease is an X-linked hereditary disorder, denoting that the α-GAL A-producing gene is situated on the X chromosome. As males possess a solitary X chromosome, this condition consequently predominantly impacts males. However, females carrying a mutated copy of the gene are also susceptible to symptoms, although the severity of which can differ considerably between carriers.

It is estimated that Fabry disease affects between 1 in 40,000 and 117,000 males. On account of the potential for delayed onset and symptom variability, the true prevalence of the condition might exceed what has been reported.

Fabry disease has the potential to impact various physiological systems, such as the gastrointestinal tract, epidermis, kidneys, heart, and nervous system. Variations in the severity and progression of the disease may be substantial, even among relatives.

Risk Factors And Causes

Mutations in the GLA gene, which encodes the instructions for generating α-GAL A enzyme, give rise to Fabry disease. As a consequence of these mutations, enzyme activity is diminished or nonexistent, causing GL-3 to accumulate in a variety of cells and tissues.

Fabry disease is an X-linked disorder, which means that males carrying a mutated copy of the gene are generally affected. Conversely, females carrying a single mutated copy may serve as carriers or manifest less severe symptoms.

Due to the inherited nature of Fabry disease, a family history of the condition constitutes a risk factor. On occasion, however, individuals may not have a familial predisposition to the disease as a result of novel mutations discovering the GLA gene.

Symptoms And Indications

Among affected individuals, the indications and symptoms of Fabry disease may vary considerably and may consist of the following:

1.   Chronic   pain,   which is   frequently characterized as acroparesthesia, or searing or prickly sensations in the hands and feet, is one of the   defining   symptoms   of   Fabry   disease. Childhood or adolescence is the typical onset age for this discomfort, which may deteriorate with time.

2. Skin manifestations: A considerable number of people diagnosed with Fabry disease develop angiokeratomas, which are characterized by   a reddish-purple rash that commonly affects the lower abdomen, pelvis, and buttocks. In addition, hypohidrosis, excessive perspiration, and heat intolerance may occur in some individuals.

3. Progressive kidney injury is a frequent complication of Fabry disease, which may ultimately result in renal failure. Involvement of the kidneys may manifest as proteinuria (urinary protein excess), hematuria (urinary blood), or impaired kidney function.

4. Cardiac complications: Cardiomyopathy (enlarged or distended heart muscle), arrhythmias (irregular heartbeats), and an increased risk of heart attack and stroke are among the cardiac complications that can result from Fabry disease.

5. Neurological manifestations: Certain individuals afflicted with Fabry disease may manifest neurological symptoms such as vertigo, hearing loss, stroke, and transient ischemic attacks (TIAs). The involvement of the central nervous system may also result in cognitive decline and psychiatric disorders.

6. Fabry disease is frequently associated with gastrointestinal complications, including abdominal pain, diarrhea, and vertigo. These manifestations are caused by the constriction of blood vessels within the gastrointestinal tract.

7. Ophthalmological manifestations: Certain individuals with Fabry disease may experience eye complications, such as clouding and corneal opacities.

It is crucial to acknowledge that the intensity and course of symptoms can differ considerably among individuals; certain individuals may encounter only a limited number of moderate symptoms, whereas others may confront substantial complications that impact multiple organs.

Analysis And Diagnosis

Fabry disease is difficult to diagnose due to its variable clinical manifestation and the symptom overlap that can occur with other conditions. Notwithstanding this, the following tests may assist in the diagnosis:

1. Blood tests are capable of quantifying the activity of the α-GAL A enzyme. Enzyme activity that is diminished is indicative of Fabry disease, although intermediate enzyme levels may be observed in some carriers.

2. Genetic testing: Molecular genetic testing can corroborate the diagnosis of Fabry disease by identifying mutations in the GLA gene. This can be especially beneficial when it comes to identifying carriers and conducting prenatal or preconception testing in families where a previous diagnosis of the condition is known.

3. Biopsy: To detect the accumulation of GL-3 deposits, a biopsy of afflicted tissues (e.g., epidermis, kidney) may be conducted in some instances; however, due to the availability of

enzyme and genetic testing, this method is utilized less frequently for diagnostic purposes.

4. Utilizing imaging modalities including computed tomography (CT) scans, magnetic resonance imaging (MRI), and echocardiography, complications and organ involvement associated with Fabry disease may be evaluated.

Intervention and timely diagnosis are crucial for the management of Fabry disease and the prevention of complications. Symptom management, supportive care, and enzyme replacement therapy (ERT), which can aid in GL-3 accumulation reduction and disease progression slowing, comprise the majority of treatment approaches.

Furthermore, specific complications such as cardiovascular problems, kidney disease, and neurological symptoms may be addressed through the implementation of lifestyle adjustments, pharmaceutical interventions, and other specialized measures. Individuals and families impacted by Fabry's disease should seek genetic counseling to deliberate on matters such as inheritance patterns, reproductive alternatives, and accessible support systems.

CHAPTER TWO

Alternatives To Treatment

Fabry disease is commonly managed through a combination of therapeutic interventions that target symptom relief, complication prevention, and disease progression inhibition. Among the most important treatment options are:

1. Enzyme replacement therapy (ERT) is a fundamental component of the management approach for Fabry disease. ERT is administered via intravenous infusion of a synthetic form of -Gal A enzyme, which aids in the degradation of Gb3 accumulation in the body. Agalsidase alfa and agalsidase beta are the two ERT medications certified for the treatment of Fabry disease.

2. Chaperone Therapy: Pharmacological chaperones, which are small molecules, are an

additional therapeutic strategy that functions by stabilizing the mutant α-Gal A enzyme. This facilitates its transportation to its intended intracellular site and enhances its overall functionality. Migalastat is an approved oral chaperone therapy for patients with Fabry disease who have amenable mutations.

3. Pain Management: One prevalent and incapacitating manifestation of Fabry disease is neuropathic pain. In addition to topical agents, physical therapy, acupuncture, and anticonvulsants, antidepressants, and anticonvulsants may be utilized in pain management strategies.

4. Fabry disease manifests in a variety of ways, with gastrointestinal disturbances, cutaneous lesions, and cardiovascular complications being just a few examples. To address these symptoms, individualized symptomatic treatments may be necessary.

ERT Is Enzyme Replacement Therapy

A significant advancement in the treatment of Fabry disease has been ERT. ERT, through the administration of exogenous α-Gal A enzyme, endeavors to diminish the buildup of Gb3 in cells and tissues, consequently mitigating symptoms and decelerating the advancement of the disease.

It is essential to note, however, that ERT does not completely reverse the damage that has already been done to organs afflicted by Fabry disease.

ERT's efficacy may fluctuate contingent upon variables including disease severity, age of treatment initiation, and the existence of particular mutations. Although ERT has demonstrated efficacy in stabilizing specific aspects of the disease and enhancing the quality of life, it may not entirely impede the advancement of complications, especially in cases that have reached an advanced stage.

Pain Management Techniques

One of the defining symptoms of Fabry disease is neuropathic pain, which has the potential to greatly diminish the quality of life for those who are afflicted. Pain management in Fabry disease frequently necessitates a multidisciplinary, patient-specific approach. Possible inclusions:

1. Pharmaceutical Interventions: Anticonvulsants (e.g., pregabalin and gabapentin), tricyclic antidepressants (e.g., amitriptyline and nortriptyline), and selective serotonin-norepinephrine reuptake inhibitors (e.g., duloxetine and venlafaxine) are among the medications that may be employed in the management of neuropathic pain.

2. Topical treatments, including lidocaine patches and capsaicin cream, have the potential to alleviate pain in particular areas of distress by acting as topical agents.

3. Physical Therapy: Stretching exercises, massage, and transcutaneous electrical nerve stimulation (TENS) are all examples of physical therapy techniques that may aid in pain relief and mobility enhancement.

4. Psychological Support: The mental well-being of individuals with chronic pain may be adversely affected, thus seeking assistance from support groups or therapists may prove advantageous in managing pain and enhancing the overall state of health.

Cardiac Difficulties

In Fabry disease, cardiac complications are a major cause for concern because they can contribute to an increase in morbidity and mortality. Cardiomyopathy, arrhythmias, left ventricular hypertrophy (LVH), and valvular abnormalities are frequent cardiac manifestations of Fabry disease. Possible cardiac complication management strategies include:

1. Consistent cardiac evaluations, encompassing electrocardiography (ECG), echocardiography, and cardiac magnetic resonance imaging (MRI), are critical in the identification and surveillance of cardiac irregularities.

2. Pharmacological interventions: To regulate hypertension, avert arrhythmias, and maintain cardiac health, pharmaceutical agents including angiotensin-converting enzyme (ACE) inhibitors, angiotensin receptor blockers (ARBs), beta-blockers, and antiarrhythmic medications may be administered.

3. Cardiac Interventions: Certain cardiac complications may necessitate cardiac interventions, including the implantation of a pacemaker, cardioverter-defibrillator, or valve replacement surgery.

4. A heart-healthy diet, regular physical activity, abstinence from smoking, and moderate alcohol consumption are examples of lifestyle modifications that can aid in the management of cardiac risk factors and the improvement of cardiovascular health as a whole.

Renal Difficulties

Renal complications are a significant facet of Fabry disease, as the progressive deterioration of the kidneys ranks among the most prevalent reasons for illness and death among those affected. Proteinuria, a decrease in glomerular filtration rate (GFR), progressive renal insufficiency, and end-stage renal disease (ESRD) are all potential renal manifestations of Fabry disease. Possible renal complications may be managed as follows:

1. Renal Function Monitoring: Consistent monitoring of renal function is critical for the timely identification and treatment of renal complications. This is achieved through the utilization of urine protein excretion, serum creatinine, and GFR estimations.

2. Regulation of Blood Pressure: Adherence to strict blood pressure management, frequently accomplished via ACE inhibitors or ARBs, is of paramount importance in mitigating the advancement of renal disease and lowering the likelihood of cardiovascular incidents.

3. Renal Replacement Therapy: Hemodialysis or peritoneal dialysis are examples of renal replacement therapy options that may be required in cases of advanced renal failure to

maintain adequate kidney function and control uremic symptoms.

4. Kidney Transplantation: Eligible Fabry disease patients with end-stage renal disease (ESRD) may be eligible for kidney transplantation, which presents the prospect of enhanced long-term survival and quality of life.

In summary, Fabry disease is an intricate pathology affecting multiple systems, necessitating a holistic and interdisciplinary strategy for its control. Although interventions for cardiac and renal complications, enzyme replacement therapy, and pain management can alleviate symptoms and improve prognoses, additional research is required to develop more effective therapies and increase our understanding of the disease. Optimal care for individuals afflicted with Fabry disease necessitates timely detection, consistent surveillance, and personalized therapeutic strategies.

Neurological Difficulties

Neurological complications are prevalent among individuals with Fabry disease and can have a substantial detrimental effect on their overall well-being. These complications are exacerbated by the accumulation of Gb3 in the nervous system, specifically in neurons and tiny blood vessels. The following are examples of neurological manifestations:

1. Peripheral neuropathy is characterized by the presence of acroparesthesia, which consists of pain and anomalous sensations in the hands and feet. The debilitating and severe nature of this neuropathic pain may result in reduced mobility and daily functioning impairment.

2. Stroke and Cerebrovascular Events: The risk of stroke and other cerebrovascular events is increased by the accumulation of Gb3 in blood vessels. In patients with Fabry, these complications

may manifest during their youth and have the potential to cause enduring neurological impairments.

3. Brain imaging studies frequently detect white matter lesions, which serve as indicators of disease affecting the small blood vessels. Cognitive impairment may result from these lesions, encompassing challenges related to attention, memory, executive function, and memory.

4. Autonomic Dysfunction: Symptoms of autonomic nervous system dysfunction may include abnormal perspiration, resistance to temperature regulation, and gastrointestinal disturbances.

5. Progressive sensorineural hearing loss is a frequent complication of Fabry disease. Hearing aids or other interventions may be necessary to enhance communication and quality of life.

A multidisciplinary approach is customary in the management of neurological complications associated with Fabry's disease. This approach encompasses pain management, stroke prevention strategies, and supportive therapies that target particular symptoms.

CHAPTER THREE

Dermatological Expressions

Fabry disease is characterized by a multitude of dermatological manifestations that result from the buildup of Gb3 in blood vessels and skin cells. These manifestations frequently manifest during childhood and may consist of:

1. Angiokeratomas are diminutive lesions characterized by dark red or purple pigmentation. They commonly manifest in regions prone to heightened irritation or trauma, including the lower abdomen, buttocks, pelvis, and thighs. While angiokeratomas are noncancerous, they may induce pruritus and distress.

2. A condition characterized by dilated blood vessels near the surface of the skin, telangiectasia manifests as diminutive, crimson veins resembling

spiders. These characteristics may manifest on the lips, face, and mucous membranes.

3. Sweating Abnormalities: Certain patients of Fabry may encounter atypical sweating patterns, such as hypohidrosis (reduced perspiration) or hyperhidrosis (excessive sweating), both of which may contribute to challenges in regulating body temperature.

4. Corneal Opacities: Gb3 deposits may also form on the cornea, resulting in visual impairment of corneal opacities.

5. Patients may potentially encounter searing or gunshot sensations in the epidermis, particularly when acroparesthesia is present.

Asymptomatic treatment is utilized in the management of dermatological manifestations to ameliorate pain and enhance the aesthetic appeal of skin lesions. Surgical excision of large or bothersome angiokeratomas, laser therapy for telangiectasia, and topical treatments for irritation may all be included.

Pediatric Fabry Disease Management

A comprehensive strategy is required to treat Fabry disease in children, which targets both the symptoms and the underlying metabolic defect. Intervention and early detection are of the utmost importance to mitigate or prevent organ harm and enhance long-term prognoses. Key elements of child management include:

1. Enzyme Replacement Therapy (ERT): The cornerstone of treatment for Fabry disease is ERT utilizing recombinant α-Gal A enzyme. Early initiation of ERT can enhance overall prognosis and impede the progression of organ injury.

2. Symptomatic treatment may be required to address particular symptoms, including but not limited to pain, gastrointestinal disturbances, and cutaneous manifestations. Medication, physical therapy, and supportive care measures may be required.

3. Regular monitoring is essential for evaluating the progression of Fabry disease in children and determining the efficacy of treatment. Clinical evaluations, laboratory analyses, imaging investigations, and specialized assessments conducted by multidisciplinary teams may be included in this process.

4. It is critical to provide children and their families with education and support to assist them in managing the difficulties associated with having a chronic genetic disorder. Genetic counseling, psychosocial support, and access to patient advocacy groups and resources are all potential components of this.

5. Ongoing investigation into novel treatment modalities and therapeutic approaches is imperative to enhance outcomes for pediatric patients afflicted with Fabry disease. This includes the development of innovative strategies for early detection and intervention, gene therapy, and novel therapeutic approaches.

To maximize outcomes and enhance quality of life, the management of Fabry disease in children necessitates a collective endeavor encompassing healthcare providers, patients, families, and researchers.

Counseling On Genetics And Family Planning

Genetic counseling is of paramount importance in the management of Fabry disease, specifically in risk assessment and family planning. The following are essential components of genetic counseling for Fabry disease:

1. Genetic counselors evaluate the likelihood that an individual or family will develop Fabry disease by considering pertinent factors such as family history, genetic testing outcomes, and genetic testing results. They furnish data about patterns of inheritance, risks of recurrence, and the probability of disease transmission to subsequent generations.

2. Individuals and couples are assisted by genetic counselors in making well-informed decisions regarding family planning, including adoption, preimplantation genetic diagnosis (PGD), and prenatal testing (PGD). A discourse ensues regarding the prospective advantages, constraints, and ethical implications that are linked to every alternative.

3. Psychosocial support is an essential component of genetic counseling, as it assists families and individuals in managing the emotional and psychological repercussions associated with Fabry's disease. This may involve confronting

emotions such as remorse, sorrow, anxiety, and future uncertainty.

4. Education and Advocacy: Genetic counselors disseminate comprehensive information regarding Fabry disease, encompassing its etiology, inheritance patterns, clinical manifestations, and treatment alternatives, to patients, families, and healthcare providers. They champion the provision of support services, medical care, and genetic testing to enhance the quality of life and overall prognosis for those impacted and their families.

5. Genetic counselors are engaged in multidisciplinary collaboration with mental health professionals, physicians, obstetricians, and medical geneticists to offer comprehensive care and assistance to families and individuals impacted by Fabry disease.

In the context of Fabry's disease, genetic counseling is of the utmost importance in enabling families and individuals to make well-informed choices regarding family planning and healthcare management.

CHAPTER FOUR

The Mental And Emotional Consequences

Affected individuals and their families may experience profound psychological and emotional effects from having Fabry disease. The potential for progressive organ injury, the chronic nature of the disease, and its unpredictable course can give rise to a range of psychosocial challenges, which may include:

1. Anxiety and depression, among other mood disorders, may become more prevalent as a result of managing a chronic genetic disorder such as Fabry disease. Anxieties regarding the advancement of disease, immobility, and the unpredictability of the future may all contribute to psychological distress.

2. Grief and loss may be encountered by individuals and families impacted by Fabry disease due to the prognosis, alterations in health conditions, and constraints imposed by the ailment. This may involve experiencing grief over the loss of independence, physical function, and plans.

3. Social isolation and loneliness may ensue for those who are afflicted with a rare disease such as Fabry, as it may be difficult to locate peers who can relate to their circumstances. Lack of awareness, stigma, and misconceptions regarding the disease may also contribute to social barriers.

4. Financial strain can be a consequence of the substantial healthcare expenditures required to manage Fabry's disease. These expenditures encompass medical care, medications, and supportive therapies, among others. A supplementary burden and tension may be

imposed on affected individuals and their families by financial constraints.

5. The development of efficacious coping strategies is critical in effectively managing the psychological and emotional repercussions associated with Fabry's disease. Potential actions to consider encompass consulting healthcare professionals for assistance, participating in patient support groups, adopting self-care strategies, and cultivating robust social support systems.

To effectively attend to the psychological and emotional requirements of individuals and families impacted by Fabry's disease, it is imperative to adopt a comprehensive strategy that combines medical, psychological, and social support services. This may encompass the provision of educational resources, counseling, psychotherapy, and peer support groups, all of which aim to foster resilience, adaptability, and holistic welfare.

Modifications To One's Lifestyle And Supportive Care

Fabry disease necessitates the implementation of specific lifestyle adjustments and the pursuit of supportive care to alleviate symptoms and enhance overall quality of life.

1. A healthy diet, which is limited in fat and sodium, is frequently recommended to patients to promote cardiovascular well-being and alleviate symptoms like gastrointestinal distress.

2. Regular, moderate exercise can aid in the maintenance of cardiovascular health, the improvement of circulation, and the management of symptoms such as muscle pain and fatigue.

3. Patients may be required to refrain from exposure to stimuli that exacerbate symptoms, including but not limited to high temperatures, tension, and specific medications.

4. Pain Management: Effective pain management is of utmost importance in enhancing the quality of life for individuals with Fabry disease, as it is a prevalent symptom. Medication, physical therapy, and complementary therapies may be required.

5. Consistent monitoring and management of complications, including but not limited to renal dysfunction, cardiovascular ailments, and neurological disorders, are critical for averting additional harm and upholding general well-being.

6. Psychological Support: The mental well-being of an individual may be significantly impacted by the challenges of managing a chronic condition such as Fabry disease. Counseling, support groups, and additional psychological interventions may prove advantageous for patients in managing the emotional difficulties that are inherent in the illness.

7. Genetic counseling can assist families and individuals in comprehending the inheritance pattern of Fabry's disease, enabling them to make well-informed choices regarding family planning and gaining access to suitable support services.

8. Consistent Medical Follow-Up: It is imperative to schedule routine appointments with healthcare professionals who specialize in Fabry disease to monitor the progression of the condition, make necessary adjustments to treatment regimens, and attend to any emergent symptoms or complications that may arise.

Insurance And Financial Considerations

Because of the requirement for ongoing medical care, medications, and supportive therapies, Fabry disease management can be expensive. Families and patients may encounter a multitude of financial obstacles, which may consist of:

1. Healthcare Expenditures: The financial burden of doctor visits, diagnostic tests, medications, and medical procedures can accumulate considerably over time. Specialized care for certain patients may necessitate the involvement of multidisciplinary teams, thereby exacerbating the financial burden of healthcare.

2. Fabry disease is conventionally managed with enzyme replacement therapy (ERT); nevertheless, this course of treatment can be quite costly. In addition, patients may necessitate pharmaceutical interventions to control symptoms and complications, including analgesics, anticoagulants, and blood pressure medications.

3. Insurance Coverage: To afford essential medications and medical care, patients must have adequate health insurance coverage. Nevertheless, coverage for uncommon diseases such as Fabry disease may differ based on the particular policy and insurance provider.

4. Financial Assistance Programs: To assist eligible patients in managing the expenses associated with medications, such as ERT, certain pharmaceutical companies provide patient assistance programs or co-pay assistance programs.

5. Disability benefits may be required for individuals with Fabry disease who are unable to work and earn a livelihood due to severe symptoms. To support their families, patients may qualify for disability benefits or other forms of financial assistance.

6. Tax Deductions: Certain nations offer tax deductions or credits to individuals with chronic illnesses, such as Fabry disease, in recognition of expenditures such as home modifications, medical costs, and other pertinent expenditures.

7. Effective financial management of the financial repercussions of Fabry disease on families and individuals requires the development of a comprehensive financial plan that takes into consideration prospective disability, long-term care requirements, and ongoing medical expenses.

CHAPTER FIVE

Support And Advocacy Groups

Advocacy and support groups are of paramount importance in increasing consciousness regarding Fabry disease, promoting enhanced availability of healthcare and treatments, and furnishing patients and their families with assistance and resources. These organizations provide an array of services, which comprise:

1. Education and Awareness: Advocacy groups endeavor to augment the comprehension and consciousness of the general public, policymakers, and healthcare professionals regarding Fabry disease.

To disseminate knowledge regarding the disease, they coordinate awareness campaigns, manage events, and distribute educational materials.

2. Patient Support: Support groups provide individuals and families affected by Fabry disease with a sense of community and connection. In addition to offering practical guidance and emotional support, they facilitate connections with others who have undergone comparable circumstances.

3. Advocacy organizations furnish comprehensive information and resources about Fabry disease, encompassing support services, treatment alternatives, clinical trials, and research progressions. Organizations may establish and manage online platforms, helplines, and peer support programs to provide information and aid patients and caregivers.

4. Advocacy Efforts: These organizations support rare disease legislation, enhanced access to healthcare, insurance coverage for treatments, and funding for research, all of which are policies and

initiatives that benefit individuals with Fabry disease.

5. Research Funding: Numerous advocacy organizations solicit funds to support fundamental science research, clinical trials, and studies on patient outcomes and quality of life about Fabry disease. Through their financial support of research endeavors, these organizations aid in the advancement of novel therapies and remedies for Fabry disease.

6. Advocacy groups foster collaboration and partnerships with various stakeholders, including healthcare providers, researchers, pharmaceutical companies, government agencies, and others, to promote the Fabry disease community's interests and enhance patient care and outcomes.

Adaptation Strategies And Life Quality

Managing Fabry's disease necessitates the implementation of coping mechanisms that encompass symptom control, emotional stability, and quality of life optimization.

1. Prioritizing self-care activities, including ensuring adequate rest, adhering to a well-balanced diet, engaging in regular physical activity, and employing relaxation techniques, can assist individuals in effectively managing stress and preserving their overall health.

2. Acquiring the ability to regulate activities and conserve energy is critical for effectively managing fatigue and preventing the exacerbation of symptoms. Regular pauses and the division of labor into more manageable components can aid in the prevention of overexertion.

3. It is advisable to establish a robust support system comprising family members, acquaintances, healthcare professionals, and fellow patients. This can offer invaluable insights, practical aid, and emotional solace while managing Fabry's disease.

4. Maintaining Knowledge: By acquiring knowledge about Fabry disease, such as its symptoms, treatments, and management strategies, individuals gain the ability to proactively advocate for their health and make well-informed decisions.

5. Establishing Realistic Objectives: By establishing realistic objectives and priorities, people can concentrate their efforts and resources on endeavors and activities that provide them with purpose and satisfaction, while also recognizing and embracing the constraints imposed by the illness.

6. It is imperative to prioritize the management of emotional difficulties, including but not limited to mourning, anxiety, depression, and social isolation, to preserve one's psychological well-being. Individuals may find it beneficial to engage in support groups, seek professional counseling, or implement mindfulness and relaxation techniques as coping mechanisms against these challenges.

7. Flexibility, resilience, and adaptation are critical qualities that individuals must possess to effectively manage the uncertainties and difficulties associated with living with a chronic illness such as Fabry disease. The acquisition of coping mechanisms and problem-solving approaches can enable people to navigate the challenges and triumphs of life with greater efficacy.

8. Prioritize Quality of Life: Despite the difficulties presented by Fabry's disease, one can augment their overall quality of life by

directing their attention towards facets of existence that elicit happiness, contentment, and fulfillment. Well-being and resilience can be enhanced through the pursuit of meaningful activities, engagement in personal interests, the expenditure of time with loved ones, and the maintenance of an optimistic mindset.

Experimental Therapies And New Therapies

Notwithstanding substantial advancements in the management of Fabry disease, innovative therapeutic approaches that tackle unfulfilled medical requirements and enhance patient prognoses remain imperative. In this regard, several emerging therapies and ongoing clinical trials exhibit promise:

1. Gene therapy is an intervention that seeks to introduce functional copies of the defective gene accountable for Fabry disease into the

organism. This is done to reinstate regular enzyme activity and inhibit the buildup of Gb3. Gene therapy for Fabry disease is currently undergoing early-stage clinical trials, and promising results have been observed in preclinical investigations.

2. Chaperone therapy utilizes small molecules known as chaperones to stabilize misfolded or dysfunctional proteins, such as the mutant α-Gal A enzyme implicated in Fabry disease. The objective of chaperone therapy is to augment the mutant enzyme's activity while facilitating its appropriate folding and operation. Clinical trials are currently examining a variety of chaperone molecules for the treatment of Fabry disease.

3. Substrate Reduction Therapy (SRT) is a therapeutic modality that targets the inhibition of precursor molecule synthesis to decrease the body's production of Gb3. The safety and efficacy of drugs that target enzymes involved in Gb3

synthesis are currently being assessed in clinical trials for the treatment of Fabry disease.

4. Concerning Fabry disease, enhanced enzyme replacement therapy (ERT): Scholars are investigating methods to enhance the therapy's stability, efficacy, and delivery. These activities encompass the creation of innovative enzyme formulations, the improvement of the properties of pre-existing enzymes through modification and the exploration of alternative routes of administration.

5. Combinatorial Therapies: The integration of various treatment modalities, including ERT, chaperone therapy, and SRT, has the potential to provide patients with Fabry disease with synergistic benefits and enhanced prognoses. Ongoing clinical trials are being conducted to assess the safety, efficacy, and potential for disease modification of combination therapies.

6. Biomarker discovery refers to the identification of quantifiable indicators that signify disease activity, progression, or treatment response. The identification of dependable biomarkers for Fabry disease may enhance the ability to diagnose the condition at an early stage, track its progression, and assess the effectiveness of treatments in clinical trials.

7. Patient-centered outcomes research endeavors to integrate the viewpoints, inclinations, and priorities of patients afflicted with Fabry disease into the process of designing and assessing clinical trials. By ensuring that interventions are by the values and requirements of both patients and caregivers, this methodology ultimately enhances patient contentment and quality of life.

8. International Collaboration It is essential that pharmaceutical companies, patient advocacy groups, clinicians, and researchers collaborate globally to advance the development and

implementation of new therapies for Fabry disease. Collaborative networks, international registries, and research consortia enable the exchange of data, the standardization of protocols, and the coordination of scientific endeavors across oceanic boundaries.

In essence, Fabry disease is an intricate hereditary condition that necessitates a comprehensive multidisciplinary approach to its management. This entails implementing coping mechanisms, advocating for patients, facilitating access to emergent therapies via clinical trials, and implementing lifestyle modifications and supportive care. A collaborative effort among policymakers, healthcare providers, researchers, and advocacy organizations can elevate the quality of life and optimize outcomes for individuals afflicted with Fabry disease by attending to the varied requirements of these individuals and their families.

CHAPTER SIX

Healthcare Group Cooperation

Collaboration among diverse healthcare professionals is of utmost importance due to the multisystemic nature of Fabry disease and the intricate management of its symptoms and complications. Fabry disease patients generally receive comprehensive care through the implementation of a multidisciplinary approach, which encompasses the expertise of various specialists including geneticists, nephrologists, cardiologists, neurologists, dermatologists, and genetic counselors.

Using this collective endeavor, comprehensive care for the patient is secured, encompassing diagnostic testing, genetic counseling, symptom management, and disease progression monitoring. Effective team coordination and communication are critical components in maximizing patient outcomes and enhancing quality of life.

Empowerment And Education Of Patients

Patient education is of the utmost importance in enabling Fabry disease patients to take an active role in their care and make well-informed decisions regarding their health. It is crucial to furnish patients and their families with precise and easily obtainable information about the characteristics of the ailment, its manifestations, possible complications, treatment options, and approaches to condition management.

Providing patients with the necessary information and abilities to effectively manage their condition can have a positive impact on treatment regimen adherence, self-care behaviors, and overall health. In addition, individuals afflicted with Fabry disease may find support groups and patient advocacy organizations to be invaluable resources. These entities provide avenues for social interaction, practical guidance, and assistance among peers.

Confronting Obstacles In The Management Of Diseases

The management of Fabry disease is a complex undertaking owing to its progressive nature and the extensive array of symptoms and complications that may ensue. Difficulties may encompass prolonged therapeutic duration, restricted diagnostic alternatives, exorbitant therapy expenses, and the requirement for continuous monitoring and administration of numerous organ systems.

Healthcare providers must employ a proactive and patient-centered approach to care to confront these challenges. This may entail proactive identification via newborn screening or genetic testing, individualized therapeutic strategies customized to the unique requirements and symptoms of each patient, availability of auxiliary resources like financial aid programs, and routine monitoring to track the advancement of the disease and modify therapy as required.

Whole-Conscious Methods Of Wellness

Complementing medical interventions that target the management of symptoms and complications associated with Fabry disease, holistic approaches to wellness may contribute to the enhancement of patients' general health and well-being.

The treatment plan may encompass lifestyle modifications such as maintaining a balanced diet, engaging in regular physical activity, employing stress management techniques, and ensuring sufficient rest.

In addition, it is critical to consider the psychosocial dimensions of coping with a chronic illness such as Fabry disease to foster psychological and emotional well-being. Facilitating patients' access to counseling, support groups, and additional mental health resources can assist them in managing the difficulties associated with their condition and sustaining a constructive perspective on life.

Integrative Medicine And Alternative Therapies

Integrative medicine approaches, which integrate evidence-based complementary therapies with conventional medical treatments, may provide patients with Fabry disease with additional benefits. These therapies have the potential to mitigate symptoms, promote holistic health and well-being, and enhance the overall quality of life.

Individuals afflicted with Fabry disease may find herbal remedies, acupuncture, massage therapy, dietary supplements, and mind-body techniques like yoga and meditation to be advantageous integrative medicine modalities. Patients must ensure that any alternative or complementary therapies they consider are safe and appropriate in light of their unique health history and conditions by consulting with their healthcare team beforehand.

Summary

In summary, Fabry disease is an uncommon hereditary disorder that exerts extensive systemic consequences, affecting a multitude of organs and physiological processes. Although infrequent, this condition has far-reaching consequences, frequently resulting in substantial morbidity and diminished quality of life for those who are impacted. The pathophysiology of the disease is distinguished by the insufficiency of the enzyme alpha-galactosidase A, which leads to the buildup of glycosphingolipids (primarily globotriaosylceramide (Gb3)) in cells across the entire organism.

Prompt identification and intervention are essential for the effective management of Fabry disease. Enzyme replacement therapy (ERT) has significantly transformed the therapeutic domain by providing symptomatic relief and potentially impeding the progression of the disease. The need for lifelong therapy, the high cost of treatment, and the variable response of patients are, nevertheless, obstacles that persist.

Investigations into alternative therapeutic approaches, including substrate reduction therapy and gene therapy, exhibit potential in mitigating these obstacles and enhancing prognoses for patients afflicted with Fabry disease. Furthermore, continuous endeavors in the realms of genetic screening and disease awareness are critical to promote opportune intervention and facilitate early detection.

The imperative for improved comprehension and control of Fabry disease necessitates the utmost importance of collaboration among healthcare practitioners, researchers, patients, and advocacy organizations. Through collaborative efforts, it is possible to advance the development of more precise diagnostics and therapies, and ultimately elevate the quality of life for individuals afflicted with this intricate ailment.

THE END